Leukemia Lessons

Maria R. Mabe

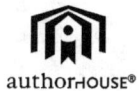

authorHOUSE®

AuthorHouse™
1663 Liberty Drive
Bloomington, IN 47403
www.authorhouse.com
Phone: 1-800-839-8640

First published by AuthorHouse 6/21/2011

ISBN: 978-1-4567-4484-7 (sc)
ISBN: 978-1-4567-4482-3 (e)

Library of Congress Control Number: 2011903986

Printed in the United States of America

Pictured on front cover: Left to right, Maria, Sara, Betty, and Susan
in October 2000 at Weber Reunion in Troy Indiana.

To my wonderful Mother,

Elizabeth Catherine Cheaney
September 6, 1943 to August 29, 2001.

...

A portion of the proceeds of this book will be donated to the
Indianapolis Chapter of the Leukemia and Lymphoma Society.

Prologue

Betty's love for God was preeminent in her life. She expressed this in her work, family, church, and friends, among whom I was privileged to be one. We were friends here on earth from 1992-2001.

Wanda Pear, LPN

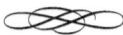

IT WILL BE 10 YEARS on August 29, 2011, since I watched my mother leave this world due to the disease Acute Myeloid Leukemia (AML). If I had tried to write this right after she left me, this book would have been filled with 100% anger. I am still 100% angry, but not 100% filled with anger. It is more sadness and missing that I am filled with now. Some days it is more, some days it is less. That is how grief goes. I lost a great person and I continue to realize her void every day. I may have taken her for granted, but I will never forget this wonderful person. I continually remind myself that she is not in pain and she is also in heaven.

I wanted to write this book to lend advice to other adult children who are on the journey of losing their parent just when the relationship turns from parent/child to friend/friend relationship. Also, I wanted to lend a perspective, as I am a health care provider (Speech Language Pathologist) who knew nothing about Leukemia when Mom was diagnosed. I also wanted to provide my nieces and nephews with a "history" of Gran Betty that they will be able to keep forever and pass on to their children.

And finally, I wanted to provide others with a summary of my leukemia lessons that I learned.

In 1993, I remember seeing teams for the Leukemia/Lymphoma Society and thinking they are just fighting a childhood exotic disease. I also thought how lucky I was that cancer had not touched my immediate family. I may have provided a donation, but never really thought about what was being fought.

Cancer did initially touch my extended family as my Aunt Alma had breast cancer surgery and successfully made it to remission around 1996. Then, my uncle, my mother's awesome brother, Tom Weber, developed colon cancer in the late 90s. My Mom who was a family practice nurse in a doctor's office began the caring relative role as Tom's sister. She was a very compassionate sister. Mom went about her way providing support to her siblings, working in a busy family practice office, and providing support to her own family. I remember thinking, "My Mom is invincible."

I will remember it clearly as long as I live. On Thursday, June 7, 1999, Mom and I were walking up the hill from the Our Lady of Greenwood Festival to the parking lot to drive home, when she said, "It is so hard to believe that we now have a family member with active cancer." Little did we know that on Friday, June 18, 1999, our lives would be forever changed when she was diagnosed with AML. Thus, adding to the number of family members with cancer.

Because I was ignorant, the clues that Mom gave did not faze me. She showed me these little bruises on her arm about a week ago before the diagnosis. She even showed my sister Sara little bruises back in mid May of '99. (The more I think about it, Mom was just in denial. She had seen these signs in her office patients and I think she was just in shock and also thought, "I am going to not be identified as 'sick with cancer', until I absolutely have to be identified.") We both brushed it off. She was very tired the week before her official diagnosis; I assumed it was because she was always the busy, caring Mom on the go, either relating to work or family.

On Sunday, June 9, 1999, we spent the day volunteering at the Our Lady of Greenwood Summer Festival selling bracelets in the ticket booth on All You Could Ride Day. Oh my. It was so hot and busy; we both could not wait to leave. When we left, we both said we were going home to take a shower and that we would talk to each other in a week. She had planned to go visit her mother (Helen Weber) and mother in law (Mary Cheaney) who were both in the same nursing home in Evansville, Indiana for the first part of the week and then coming back to Indianapolis on Thursday night so she could work Friday as a nurse at Greenwood Family Practice.

The week was busy and hot. On Friday, June 18, I came home from work to pull weeds in my back yard, and had just come in side when my Dad called. "Hi Maria, I just have to call you to tell you that your Mom has been diagnosed with Leukemia." My first thought was, "Cancer!!!" I told him he was a liar. I was sobbing hysterically. How did this happen?? I just saw her last week. He patiently listened to me and said, "I hate to let you go, but I have to make more phone calls."

I did not know what to do. I called a girlfriend just to cry on the phone. She did not know what to do except to say she was sorry. I was so glad for that girlfriend to just be on the phone while I cried.

I then called one of my Mom's co-workers, Anita. I told her I couldn't believe it. She came over to give me a hug. I remember saying, "Everything has changed now." She said, "Yes it has, but she is still your mother." Anita, earlier in the day, had gotten word that Mom's boss, Dr. Richert, demanded that she go get a stat blood test at St. Francis Hospital after showing him her bruises. She wanted to wait until Saturday to get a blood test as she was off work that day. He would not hear it. After the test, she drove back to work and started working again. Dr. Richert got the call from the lab that Mom's blood count was 245,000. Normal is between 5 and 10 thousand. He grimly told her she more than likely had leukemia. He sent her to Dr. Mary Lou Mayer whose office was next to Community South. Dr. Mayer explained to Mom that she could treat her or that she could be referred to IU as she refers about 10 cases a year to Dr. Larry Cripe. Mom decided to go to Indiana University

(IU). Mom tried to call Dad at work, but the number was not right. Dr. Mayer asked where he worked, and Mom said Indianapolis Power and Light. Dr. Mayer smiled and said, "My husband works there. " (He has a different last name) Dr. Mayer got on the phone and within a few minutes Mom was talking to Dad. Talk about a small world.

Friday evening, Anita offered to take me to see her but I said, "No, we should let her rest." I think I was so shocked I could not face her yet. My Mom's friend told me I needed to get some rest. I slept fitfully, but soon it was morning. Life goes on even with a cancer diagnosis. Laundry had to be done on Saturday morning.

It was early morning when I called my Aunt Marian Seib venting my anger. She was sympathetic, but said we have to pull it together and start praying to St. Jude. I remembered about St. Jude Hospital, but I remembered thinking that it was a children's hospital and only little children get leukemia.

I finally got the nerve to call my Mom at Indiana University Hospital. I called information and was immediately dispatched to the room. The conversation went like this:

"Hi Mom ."

"Hi honey."

"I can't believe it, Mom."

"Listen, honey, I am not going to hold back the tears." She proceeded to cry. I told her she had every right to cry.

I asked if I could come see her and she asked if I would wait until Sunday so she could look a little better. She said something about being hooked up to a Leukophoresis Machine on Friday evening, and she was tired, plus, now she had a port in her chest, and she wanted one more day to rest before I came with my sister Susan to visit.

She also told me that on Friday night a doctor came to see her late that evening and she was not impressed that she could smell traces of alcohol on his breath. "Some big time physician doing Friday night visits after a cocktail party," she said. She and I both just laughed.

I said, "Okay, we will wait until Sunday." My sister Susan McDowell who lived in Bloomington at the time decided to come see me on Saturday and spend night and we would go with Dad to see Mom on Sunday. (Susan could not believe Mom was diagnosed with Leukemia, just that previous Thursday evening, Mom helped her make copies for her teaching lesson at Kinko's.) Susan was a Teaching Assistant at Indiana University, teaching beginning German while obtaining a MAT in German.

I talked to my Mom's beloved sister Elaine. She was stunned and said she would have to process this before coming up from Evansville, Indiana. I really felt for her. Elaine was one of Mom's biggest cheerleaders. She left her comfort zone and would drive up from Evansville to the IU Hospital Campus. She'd tell me that she would drive somewhat slow, people would pass her, and she would wave and say, "Go ahead and pass me, I am having a bad day." When Mom lost her hair, Elaine was even able to get Mom a free hat from J.C. Penny's. You would laugh if you knew Aunt Elaine. She said she went to Penny's and got overwhelmed by the hats.

The woman who was helping her listened to Elaine tell her about her sister. The woman gave her the hat as a gift. It was a cute blue jean hat, with a yellow flower on top.

I talked to Uncle Tom (Mom's brother) and Aunt Mary. They were very encouraging. Uncle Tom said, "I talked to my oncologist in Louisville and he said this type of blood cancer was beatable." I did not realize then that so many subtypes of AML existed. Mom had a very severe subtype of AML.

When Susan came later on Saturday, we were both irritable and tired. We made plain angel food cupcakes to take to hospital so Susan could celebrate her birthday with Mom on June 20th.

We were basket cases the whole day preparing to see Mom the next day. We argued over silly things. I had no patience. We literally fell into bed that night. I secretly dreaded going to the big IU hospital.

I had never been to IU hospital, but I had always associated it with big time medical problems and I knew this was a big time medical problem. Before going to see Mom, we went to mass with Dad at Our Lady of Greenwood. I told the news to Fr. Kneuven, and he said, "Betty Cheaney has blood cancer???"

As we were in the lobby of the hospital with Dad he approached the elevator and said we are going up to 5 North, which I would thereafter refer to in my own thoughts as 5 Hell.

As we got to the nursing station, I saw flowers on the desk. The receptionist said, "Oh these are the patient's flowers. You know, they can't have flowers in their room." I thought to myself, "What? No flowers?" Flowers are supposed to brighten the room and make a sick person feel cheerful.

All of a sudden, we opened a door and walked into a hallway. It was a stark white hallway. I thought, "This is so scary." All of a sudden I saw her name on the door, "Oh, this is really official when you see your loved ones name on the door." I looked in and saw this very tiny room, what I would later refer to as jail cell. She was sitting in a chair with her gown on with a tube hooked into her chest. This was a port. I about died. I had never seen a tube in the neck. I had seen a naso gastric tube and a feeding tube and a breathing tube, but not this tube. It was hooked up to a pole with a bag of blood that she was receiving.

She saw us and immediately said, "Hi" and then tried to start singing Happy Birthday to Susan. She cried the whole way through. I looked at her not knowing what to do. The nurse who was in the room said, "Go on in the room, give her a hug. She won't break; she won't break."

But, before we were allowed to go in, we were on the other side of the window where you have to wash your hands, put a gown on, gloves and a mask. Every time you go in to see her. I again about died; "You have got to be freaking kidding. She is really in isolation." Now, granted, I had worked with patients in isolation, but this was my own family member.

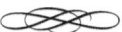

If I had a dollar for every time I wore a gown glove mask, I would be a billionaire. Boy, did I hate the ritual. However, I knew it had to be done. I forgot just once, and the nurse gently but firmly reminded me.

The room she was in was so tiny. The only items in the room: One bed, chair, T.V., a sink, a trash can, and a bedside commode.

"What? No shower? No regular toilet? You have got to be freaking kidding me." She said it was all for infection control rules. "Whatever," I thought. Mom was so mad that the wastebasket did not have a lid on it. "This is so gross," she said. (At one of Mom's later hospital stays, a nurse went out and bought her a plastic trash can with a lid on it) That did not bother me, what bothered me was the lack of decor in the room. Working as a speech therapist in rehab hospitals or just regular hospitals, the rooms were so pretty. Also, the fact that she could not have any stuffed animals in the room, only cards and pictures was sobering.

We tried to make small talk, but she was in pain even though she tried to hide it. Susan, an awesome flute player, brought her flute to play Mom a song. She played, and I guess the next-door neighbor banged on the wall to quit. I was like, "Who cares? We are trying to make our Mom feel better."

We stayed about two hours when it was clear she needed to rest. So, we went home. I fell in bed emotionally exhausted at 5 p.m. This was the worst day of my life. (Little did I know there would be a few of those worst days). I literally slept until 6 a.m. the next morning.

I was a basket case at work as I tried to tell a co-worker about the events of the previous day. As soon as work ended I made my way to the hospital. When I got to the lobby I freaked. I had no idea where I was going. I could not remember where I was the day before. I could not believe as I have an excellent memory; I felt so intimidated by the hospital. I never felt intimidated by a hospital before, but this was the big house.

I finally looked at a nurse in the hallway and trying to talk while fighting back tears I said, "Look, my Mom has leukemia, what floor is that?" She said, "Honey, 5 North."

I went right up and to the room. Not a good sight. She was in pain and she was bleeding profusely around the port. I could not believe the blood, it was like she had a gunshot wound and nobody could stop the blood. She was not with it at all. I just stared, mortified.

Our neighbors came to visit and she remarked she remembered seeing her Dad who had leukemia bleeding immensely from the port.

I went to the little lounge that seats four people. There was a woman sitting in the small room. I just cried trying not to be heard. She came over and gave me a hug. I did not know her but that hug was needed. The little lounge on 5 North may have been tiny and impersonal, but it was a refuge at times to get away from the chaotic atmosphere that sometimes existed in her room.

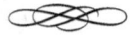

I came back to her room and it was time for Dad and I to go. Mom was not with it and the nurses told us to go home and rest. As we walked out with our neighbors, we thanked God for the warm evening. For me, it is always easier to deal with adversity when the weather is good.

From June 18 through July 15, '99, Mom was basically in a coma. Everyday I came she never woke up.

She finally aroused on July 15th. She could not believe she had been out of it. She was not happy to see all of her hair gone. We cut it all off in the hospital while she was sleeping, because she was shedding so much from the chemo and it was always making her bed messy. My sisters and I had no qualms about changing her bed or rubbing her body with lotion. We were just trying to keep her comfortable. We even argued quietly amongst each other about how much lotion to put on.

We would have whispering shouting matches with our masks on. It was funny. No way did we want to argue in front of Mom, but we were going to argue. Mom finally started to do her own self-care with help of a physical therapist and an occupational therapist on July 16th. She was proud that she could brush and comb her hair, brush her teeth and try to walk.

She announced she was ready to go home.

So, on my 32nd birthday, July 17th, she came home. She could barely walk into the room. She plopped into an easy chair. Ahh, to be home. The house was decorated in *Welcome Home!* signs courtesy of her wonderful next door neighbors, The Zabel Family. She kept saying how awesome it was to be home.

She did not get to go to her first grandchild's baptism the next week. Colin was born on May 7th, '99. Mom, Dad, and I went to see him for the first time about a week after he was born. During the Baptism, Aunt Mary stayed with her. She was disappointed, but she knew she could not go. I felt so cheated that she could not share in this special day with family. It was her first grandchild being baptized into the Catholic Church. However, I did remind myself that she did see Colin a few weeks after his birth and she held him a long time.

I took her back to Dr. Cripe's office three days after her discharge. He was such a wonderful man. I liked to think of him as Jesus walking on Earth. He was so compassionate and patient with patients and family members. He talked to us and then said, "We hope the chemo works," and made the sign of the cross. I about fell off the chair. It was refreshing to see a doctor demonstrate his Christianity. He said Mom was in partial remission. I thought, "Partial remission? That's like saying partially pregnant. Either you are or you aren't." Oh well, that is just oncology lingo.

The next few weeks, we kept thinking, "Let's stay out of the hospital as long as we can. Let's pray, eat, and have a good time." Mom did some funny things like get up in the middle of the night to eat cream puffs that Julie (the German Exchange student next door) had made. Mom barely ate the weeks of her first hospitalization. I laughed so hard when I saw her standing with the refrigerator door open and shoving a cream puff in her mouth a few nights after being home from hospital.

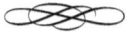

She also spent time sleeping and she had to start saying no. My Mom was the best RN in a doctor's office in the entire world. My Mom never turned her back on those in need. This sweet elderly woman called from her home to Mom's home to see if she could call in their prescriptions. She had me tell this lady she could not come back to work and she would have to let the girls at the office call in her scripts. That was hard for Mom. She gave the best allergy shots at the office and visited elderly friends at their home if they could not get out when they were sick. Mom had to quit working as nurse on 6/18/99, but she was always a nurse in her mind. I would visit at the hospital and she would say you have to get home before it really storms. I would get home and she would call in a very inaudible weak voice, "Did you get home okay?" Always the nurse. Another time, she would ask her nurse, "Don't you think she should leave now?" I would not want to and the nurse could just see me tearing up and say, "I am not getting in the middle of this." I wanted to be there for Mom at 100%, but she knew I needed my rest.

During that time, I tried to do fun things with friends. I went to an Indians game and there I met a girl who was raising money for the

Leukemia and Lymphoma Society.. When she heard my story, she kept grabbing her chest saying this is painful to hear as her Mom died from leukemia ten years earlier at Methodist Hospital. I kept thinking, "Get a grip girl. It's not that painful and my Mom ain't dying." How naive I was too think it was not painful and she would not succumb to the disease.

It was around Sept of 1999 when one evening, Mom showed me these bumps on her forehead. We thought it was acne. She went to the dermatologist, Dr. Barb Sturm who gave her all of these free samples. Mom had made referrals to her through the doctor's office so they knew each other well. I laughed when I saw the bag.

Well, IU did not laugh when she told them about the bumps. She had to get a biopsy of the bumps at an outpatient site on the IUPUI campus. She got directions and drove herself. I will never forget hearing Dr. Cripe's nurse, Pat Kneebone, tell us the bumps were probably leukemic cells and she needed to be examined immediately. What a bummer.

She was in hospital from around middle of September to the middle-to-end of October of '99. I felt so bad when I called her one day from work. It was a beautiful sunny day. She could barely talk. I told her I would take her to Brown County when she got better. She said there was no way could she go now.

I will never forget when I came to the house that Friday in October of 1999, when she had been home for an hour and she was at the kitchen table arranging family pictures in frames. She had to do something where she felt in control. What a good sight. I just hoped she did not cut her finger on the glass of the picture frames.

Mom's disease was manageable from then until March of 2000 before requiring another hospitalization. During the time of wellness, she went with me to a Neil Diamond concert in December of 1999 and she was also with her 91 year-old mother when she passed away in a nursing home in December of '99. She was so happy to be with Grandma at the end. It was bittersweet because Uncle Tom was having surgery in

11

Kentucky and could not come to Grandma Weber's funeral. He, over the phone, recommended readings to be read at her funeral. Mom looked so pretty at Grandma's funeral. She had a black velvet dress that looked good with her short hair wig.

In March of 2000, I went with Mom to the doctor. We were on cloud nine going into the appointment, because she looked so good. Everyone in the waiting room commented on how cute her curly hair was. It was straight but came back in ringlet curls after chemo. She had her blood sample taken and we waited for the doctor.

Dr. Cripe comes in the room with his shoulders slumped. "I hate to tell you this, but your counts are not good." I was so shocked, I started to cry. Mom tried to tell me to not get upset. I felt I can get upset if I want. I only thought about going back to 5 North for me as a caregiver and her as the patient.

He said, "Since this is Wednesday, I want you to wait until Monday to come in to get started so my staff can be bright eyed and bushytailed." It was going to be Easter weekend and he preferred that we wait until after Easter and come in on Monday. Who can enjoy the holiday when you know that you have to go back to 5 North? The staff at 5 North was excellent. You never knew they were having a bad day. They were the ultimate jokesters, and cheerleaders. It was just the building that stunk. Prison buildings have to be decorated prettier. The staff made 5 North the great place it was, not the building itself. I was very excited when The Simon Cancer Center was built. I thought a plaque should go on the New Hematology Unit that said, *In memory of all those who dealt with Five Hell.*

We ended up going out to eat in Franklin for Easter. It was fun, but we were teary thinking of the unknown. After arriving home from Easter Dinner, Our neighbors, The Zabel's, came over with their little kids and Mom and I were just sitting at the table boo-hooing. The neighbor took me on a walk while the kids cheered up Mom.

Kids can be so funny. A couple of days earlier when Mom told the little girl across the street that she had to go back to the hospital, (all the neighborhood kids called my Mom Miss Betty), the little girl asked, "Miss Betty, Are they going to give you new hair?" I about wet my pants. We both laughed for a while, before she gently explained the reason for going back.

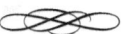

Mom went in the hospital from March to May of 2000. It was hard to visit her there on Mother's Day and not cry. It is very hard not to show your emotions in front of family members. I remember just get all of these holidays over so I don't have to think about her not being home. Mother's Day was special because Uncle Tom (who was feeling better) and Aunt Mary came to visit Mom and conducted a little prayer service. It was very soothing.

In May of 2000, I walked by myself in my first Mini Marathon. After both Grandma Weber and Grandma Cheaney died in December of '99, I thought I needed to get involved in something to take my mind off of the loss. Mom was in the hospital that weekend. I remember finishing the Mini and after resting a bit, I made the slow trek to the hospital. I came through the isolation hallway and Mom was walking with Dad along with the IV pole, wearing a mask. She said, "Oh, you look as bad as I feel." I laughed. She was worried about my sunburn. Always the nurse.

It was also hard to visit at IU because you have to pay to park. I am so glad I did not calculate how much I spent on parking. It would have made me sick to think the money I spent could have been given to charity or spent on myself.

Caring for someone while they are in the hospital is a big sacrifice. If you work your full time job and then you have another full time job dumped on you that you don't draw a paycheck from, it can be overwhelming. You only receive gratitude, which is priceless, but you do feel like it sucks the life out of you. That's when prayer comes in very handy.

June, July, August, September, and October seemed fine. We had an awesome Weber Reunion in Troy, Indiana in September of 2000. By early November, her blood counts got bad.

She was going to go in a couple weeks before Thanksgiving and start an experimental drug Mylotarg that was supposed to not knock the socks off of her. She would be home for Thanksgiving. But Mylotarg knocked her for a loop. She was ticked. "They told me it would not be that bad." I was ticked. She did not get to go home for Turkey Day. I put the turkey in as family came to celebrate. We all felt gipped that she was not there. It was also her 34th Wedding anniversary on Thanksgiving Day. It was hard to be upbeat when I visited her Wednesday night before Thanksgiving. She gave me last minute advice on dinner. It was the first time putting a turkey in all by myself.

I went to church on Thanksgiving morning and just cried. I felt robbed that Mom could not come home. A lady at church told me to quit feeling sorry for myself and make sure dinner was good for everyone. Mark, Tracy, and Colin, as well as Aunt Alma and Uncle John came for Thanksgiving and contributed to the meal. Some family ate dinner and then went to the hospital. I stayed at Mom and Dad's the entire day.

I was glad to get Thanksgiving over. In retrospect, I wished I had been more thankful.

She stayed in the hospital until December 11, 2000. She came home for two days before going back in with an infection. She would stay then until New Years Eve. We finally said, "Please let her go." "We don't want to watch football and the New Years Parade at 5 North." "The tiny little lounge?" "Come on." I did do something good for myself on Christmas Day. I made my own new tradition on Christmas Eve. I came over early to the hospital-spent the day with her and then went to mass at IU. No way was I going to my hometown church. I could not stand to see happy families together at church when Mom was stuck at IU. It was a very peaceful service as everybody there had a family member in the hospital or was an employee. As family members at IU, we were all in the club no one wanted to join.

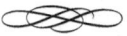

She came home New Year's Eve. It was the best present. We ate vegetable soup Susan had made. Mom left the tree up through February because she was robbed of Christmas.

She had a setback in mid January of 2001. She could barely walk into the hospital when going for a bi-weekly visit for blood counts. They had to get a wheelchair to wheel her from the car to the unit. I felt sorry for my sister Susan who had to witness this. I knew it was scary.

I think they thought she was not going to make it, because Dr. Cripe spent a lot of time with her that day.

He even said it was close to end. He wanted to admit her; she said "No way! You have had me. I am gong home," she said. He said, "Well, then, you have to come back every day for at least 2 weeks." Mom's response- "So, I've got people to bring me. Who wants to keep coming back to that old 5 North building? The people may be awesome but the setting stinks." (Thank the Lord that the Simon Cancer Center was built in 2008!!!) She did come back every day for two weeks. "I'll show them, she thought."

In the meantime, her brother, our beloved Tom Weber at age 60 was losing his battle with colon cancer in Troy, Indiana. My cousin Jen and I drove to Troy to see him at home in hospice in early February. As we were telling him good-bye, he said, "Tell her I will be waiting for her in heaven." That was very comforting to me knowing that they could be together in heaven and at the same time, devastating. He left this Earth and entered his eternal reward on February 15, 2001.

We went to his funeral in what was the coldest day in Troy. Freezing. I could not believe how calm Mom was being at a funeral home when she probably knew deep down she was going to be here soon in the casket. She even stood outside for the burial. It was so cold our tears froze on our faces.

As we got home from the weekend, we found out Dale Earnhardt had been killed in an accident. I think it was just a reminder that we all are going to die at sometime and in some manner. Mom's health improved when she got home from Uncle Tom's funeral.

She anxiously awaited the arrival of her second grandchild, Alma Elizabeth, who was born on May 28, 2001.

Susan would bring the baby home for three weeks when the baby was only 3 weeks old on June 19, 2001. Our cousin Laura was being married on June 23, 2001, and Susan wanted to be there with the baby. This was pre 9/11 and Susan relayed to me that Mom was standing by the entrance of those arriving from the plane. Susan, Manfred, and Alma were the last to get off the plane. People saw Mom and said, "Oh, you must be the excited Grandma!" Mom was smiling from ear to ear.

We all forgot she was sick. She forgot she was sick. She went to Conner Prairie for Symphony on the Prairie with Susan and little Alma, showed Alma off to family friends, took a trip to Troy, Indiana to visit Mary with Susan, Manfred and the baby. She took the baby to the doctor's office, (her former place of employment), to weigh the baby. They told her they were insulted that she thought she had to ask to weigh the baby. Mom was always respectful. She had also weighed a lot of babies at the office. Kids loved her at the office. One boy nicknamed her Dr. Betty.

Two days before, Susan left on July 25th, my brother Mark, his wife Tracy, and their son, Colin, age 2, came to see Susan, Manfred, and baby Alma. We had a great visit! Mom was even down on the floor staking poker chips with Colin. July 25th, 2001 was bittersweet when Susan, Manfred, and Alma went back to Northern Ireland. Mom and Dad were invited to a wedding of Sara's former high school boyfriend. She said, "We are going so we have something fun to do and don't have to think about little Alma not being in Indiana any more."

Mom went back to the hospital on August 1st and that day was very bitter. I came over like I usually did after work to hear about her doctor's visit. She had her bi-weekly blood test and they gave her the bad news that nothing more could be done. Her counts had skyrocketed. He told her she would have to come up with a miracle on her own. They were out of answers.

She said, "Let's go into the kitchen and call Sara." She wanted me to listen. She proceeded to tell Sara that they told her she was dying. I was shell-shocked. I started to scream. She looked very disapprovingly at me. I just could not believe it. We can put a man on the moon but we can't cure leukemia. Amazing.

She apologized to Sara. She was apologizing? She did not need to apologize for anything. I should be apologizing for being insensitive at times, saying hurtful things, being frustrated. That woman should have people apologizing to her everyday. Sorry for the insurance mix-ups, sorry you have to leave your kids soon, sorry you can't have fun with your grandkids longer, sorry you can't enjoy the fruits of your retirement. Doesn't that sound like what all terminally ill people should be hearing? Terminally ill people are brave, saintly, patient, and loving souls who care about the loved ones that they have to leave behind.

After she hung up with Sara, she said that we needed to go to Weight Watchers. I laughed and thought, "You are dying, and we are going to Weight Watchers." We had started that program together in May as cousin Laura was getting married in June and Sara was getting married in October. Mom wanted to see that I stuck with it. How saintly of her. We did go and I cried through the entire thing. The woman at the weigh in could not understand why I had tears. My Mom just told her I was having a bad day.

We then left to go eat a meal and then went to Hobby Lobby to look at shower invitations for Sara's upcoming bridal shower in September. Sara's wedding was October 20, 2001. Would she be there in person or in spirit? I had a sinking feeling the whole time I was there. I just could not believe I was losing her. I know I was selfish because she was going to get to go to heaven and be free from pain. But, I was thinking of myself and not her.

Sara's wedding at the Naval Academy was going to be beautiful Mom said. Just the previous year, Mom, Dad, and her sister Elaine along with her husband Jerry took a fall road trip to see the Academy as well as D.C. Mom and Elaine had investigated wedding dates for Sara. Mom even called Sara about an open date in 2001. They saw the chapel, both standing in silence in awe of its beauty.

On a Monday, August 27, she was told it would be over soon. She and Dad decided to go to G. H. Herrman to make funeral arrangements. Mom said, "Do you think we need an appointment?" Dad said, "Let's just go and see what they say." She courageously went to the funeral home and made out all the arrangements with Dad. A friend later told me that the employee at the funeral home could not believe how calm she was. I believe she was at peace and resigned to the fact that the battle was about over.

When I got to the house on that Monday she said that it was too pretty to be inside and was not going to a block of rooms on the other side of the isolation unit that was deemed Hospice. Hospice seemed unreal, as she was up walking around and fully alert. We went to five thirty mass at Our Lady of Greenwood and I cried through the entire mass. It was a day I will never forget, as it was the last day that Mom, Dad, and I worshipped together. It was gut wrenching. We came back to eat outside on the patio. She ate all three meals on that patio from June 1 through August 28, 2001. She and Dad had moved from our big family home for 20 some years to a small home that was easier to manage. I wish I could have videotaped her at those meals. She was happy eating at that outside table. I could see Mom really could not eat because of the sores in her mouth, but she was outside, enjoying the beautiful weather on her deck.

I sat with Mom on the front porch hugging her before I left to go home. She gave me a hug and said she was at peace with everything, but she was worried about me. I was not showing her that I would be okay. I would later feel bad about this. I had to work all day on the 28th, (No, she did not want me to call in sick to be with her). We made plans to see each other in the evening on August 29th.

At 4:00 a.m. on August 29, I received a call from Dad that awoke me from a dead sleep. "She's gone!!" She had a stroke at home and is now at Methodist Hospital in the ER. She is on a vent but will be taken off when you and Mark get here. I called Mom's friend, Anita, to drive me. She lived very close to me. I was too shaken to drive. Anita and I got a little lost on the way to IU. Subconsciously, I believe we did not want to go, we did not think it was time. Is anyone ever ready? Is it better to lose someone suddenly or watch them go through a battle? No one answer is right.

I went into the room, her eyes were open, but she was on the ventilator. I held her hand and talked to her, saying, "I am sorry this is happening." We had a great life together. Dad, myself, Mom's friend Anita, and I were in room, when her heart gave out. The breathing tube was pulled. That was the worst feeling in my life. My heart was broken. Several priests had come as well as some of Mom's other friends. I felt bad that Mark arrived from Chicago after she died. They let us keep her awhile in the ER before she had to be moved. Dad, Mark, and I came home. Mom's friend Anita had already been to the house, and cleaned up Mom and Dad's bedroom, and had bought food for us to eat for lunch. We also had a catnap before going to funeral home to set a funeral time.

The woman at GH Herrman told me, "Oh, you look just like your Mom." I sobbed.

The visitation was gratifying as Mom had a great turnout. I found a sweatshirt of hers that said, "Behind every good doctor is a GREAT NURSE." This was hung on display as well as many family pictures. The funeral was beautiful. The best songs played/sung were *On Eagle's Wings* and *Whatsoever You Do.*

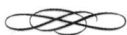

This next part I hope is helpful. When Mom was first diagnosed, I went to Border's trying to find a book on how to cope with Leukemia. I did not find it. I just learned some lessons during the illness and after.

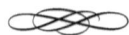

So what lessons did I learn?

Oncology medical Professionals at University Hospital in Indianapolis are the greatest. They are the most compassionate souls who have a tough job. They follow a patient to their death more often than see them through the cure. They befriend clueless families who lash out at them, blame them, and are impatient with them. They worked in an old building like 5 North, but you never knew it as they acted liked they worked at the Ritz Carlton. They always had smiles on their faces and you never knew they were having a bad day. God Bless them.

Patience is needed. This process is a marathon rollercoaster that does not end until the end is the end. You have to go with the flow as unexpected turns of events happen. If you don't go with the flow, you can get very stressed.

Special friends are needed to be with the patient/family during the process. Yvonne Sheek from Our Lady of Greenwood spent a lot of time behind the glass praying for Mom, cheering her up, and providing support to our family. Mom's friend Ellen McGee would invite Mom over for dinner after a stressful Doctor's appointment. Shirley would always have a motivational devotion to give to Mom. Anna and Jan at work would always be lifting Mom's spirit. At Christmas of '99, Mom even decorated the doctor's office for Christmas. She was touched when Dr. and Mrs. Richert sent her a gift card thanking her for their efforts. I was thankful Mom was able to decorate the office because it made her feel like she was still part of an office that she had to leave suddenly. Mom's nursing friends even had a sweatshirt that they all wore which said, "We may not have it all together, but together we have it all."

Humor is needed. I needed to have more humor during the process. I did not display much. I was always serious. Mom and I didn't see the humor in the situation when she was hospitalized. Sometimes Mom did funny things, which made me really nervous. When Uncle Tom could not go see Mom because he did not want to catch anything because of his cancer, he brought his little granddaughter Rebecca to visit outside. He called Mom on his cell phone. Mom opened up the curtains and started jumping up and down waving as Tom and Becca were jumping up and down waving. I about died because I thought the tube from the port was going to get pulled out. I would gently say, "Stop jumping." I was so scared that tube would get pulled out.

Encourage your terminal loved one do what they want to do. Sara was in her sorority sister's Mary's, wedding downtown at St. John's. While, not in the hospital, I told Mom she should not go as she could catch something landing her back in the hospital. She said, "I will sit in the last pew at St. John's with a mask on."

I didn't need to be such a killjoy.

I needed better nutrition as a family member. I was ragged because I should have taken better care of myself. I used to eat M & M's from behind the mask when I visited Mom to comfort myself. Not a good thing. I skimped on sleep and on eating and by the third evening I would be in bed as soon as I got home from work. I needed to pace myself in this marathon.

Grief support groups are priceless. I learned so much. I attended one group meeting with Mom during the two years of her illness, and went to two different sessions after her death. The support group from the Leukemia Society, that Mom and I attended, was great. When my sister Susan was in town, she came. The retreats after Mom's death were a Daughter's Without Mothers group, through St. Vincent Hospice and a Grieving Retreat through the Catholic Church.

Ongoing counseling does help. I attended counseling for 10 or 11 years starting after Mom was diagnosed. It really helps. Don't be ashamed if you need help. One can not go through this alone.

Prayer needs to be ongoing to help you get through the process. And asking for others to pray is encouraged.

Volunteering for the Leukemia Lymphoma Society does help as it gives you a chance to encourage someone else who is going through what you went through. You feel like you are doing something. But you have to volunteer when you are ready. I did not volunteer for the first year after because I was angry and I thought, I volunteered for two and a half years of her illness, I don't need to do it now. But, I started after Mom's first year anniversary of her death. It is rewarding when you see other family members volunteering in memory of a loved one. It is also rewarding seeing a family walk during the Light the Night Walk in memory of their loved ones. The family of LeAnn Cox, had a great procession during the Light the Night Walks. I read once where someone verbalized, "You can hate the world, or make the world a better place after a loved one dies." This quote was from a father who had lost his beautiful daughter to a drunk driver. I chose to make the world a better place.

Being involved in Team and Training does help you work through grief. My sister Sara did the Lava Man Triathalon in Hawaii in April of 02 raising over 5,000 dollars. I did the Mini Marathon in Indianapolis through Team in Training raising almost 2,000 dollars in 2006.

Life does go on and that person is always in your heart. Talking out loud to that person is acceptable. I would do it in privacy, as observers would think you are loony. But, then again, whatever works. Sara's wedding did go on in October of 2001, and I did talk to Mom all the time to get us through this day.

In summary, my Mom was a wonderful Christian woman. She exuded grace. I know she is in a better place and is still in her nursing role as she comforts little children in heaven who are missing their parents and also men and women who have sacrificed for their country in war, having come to heaven too soon leaving behind friend and family. 9/11 happened a little less than a month after her death. After 911, a good friend sent me a sympathy card that read, "Your mother would not want to come back to this world even if she could."

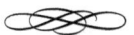

Epilogue

It is now late 2010. Sara a Naval OB Nurse Mid Wife/ Nurse Practitioner married to Dave has 4 children, Catherine, age 7, Carolyn age 5, Anthony age 3, and Mathew, 4 months old. Mom's spirit truly lives on in this family.

Susan, married to Manfred, has 3 children, Alma age 9, Hugh 7, and Alex age 5. Susan is studying to be a Mid Wife. Again, Mom truly lives on in this family.

Mark, a computer software executive, married to Tracy in 1997, now has 3 boys, Colin 11, Devin 9, and Liam, age 5. Again, Mom's spirit lives on in this family.

I married Greg in 2007. We are Super Aunt and Uncle. Mom's spirit lives on in our family.

My Dad married a wonderful lady, Cathy, in 2008. His life has truly been extended by meeting Cathy. Mom's spirit lives on in Dad as he interacts with us kids in life.

Acknowledgements

Special thanks to all of our extended family, friends, and Indiana University Medical Center Staff who supported us during Mom's illness. Special Thanks to all of our extended friends, family, and Medical Staff who have supported us these last 10 years as we have learned to cope with the loss of Betty.

Thank you to Marcella Kates for her help on this book.

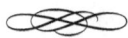

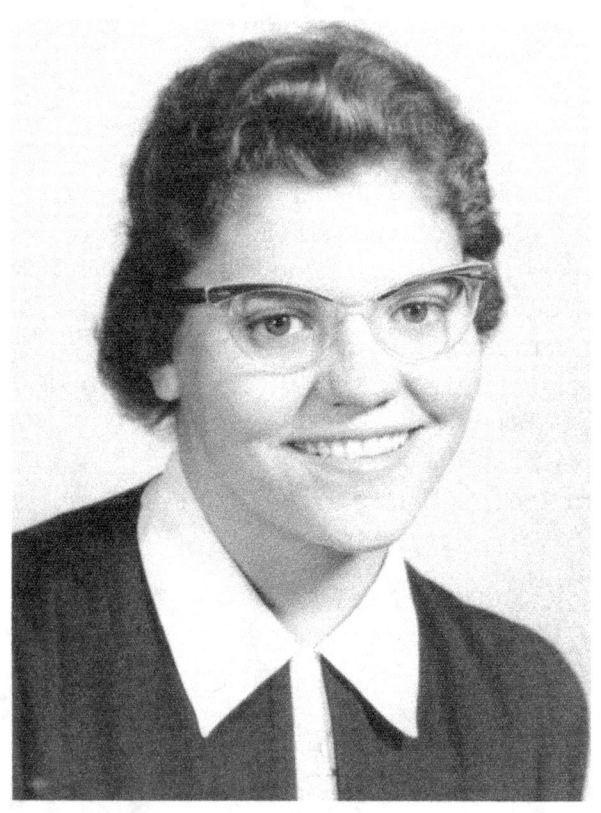

Betty Cheaney Mater Dei High School,
Evansville Indiana Class of 1961

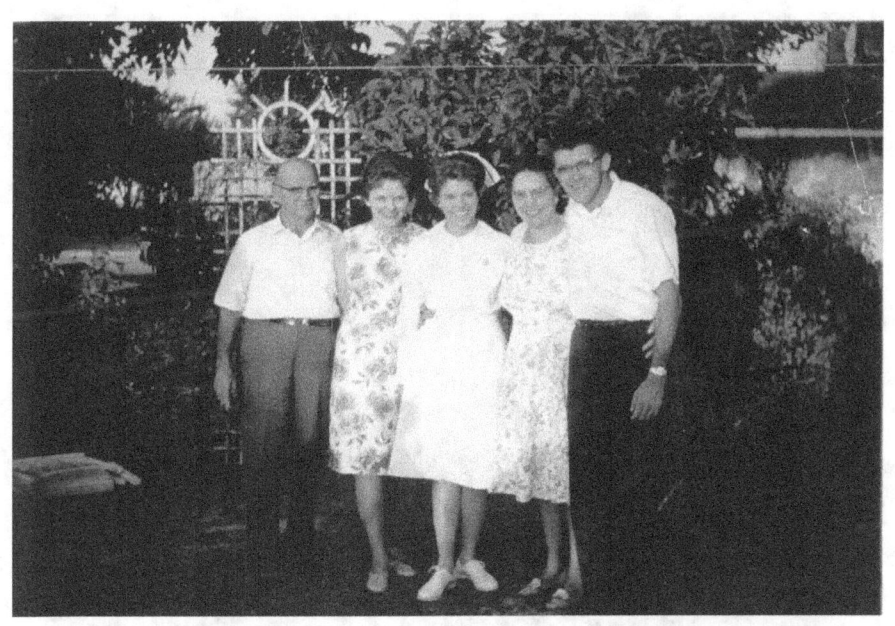

Mom's graduation from St. Mary's School of Nursing in 1964.
Grandpa Weber, Aunt Elaine, Mom,
Grandma Weber, and Uncle Tom

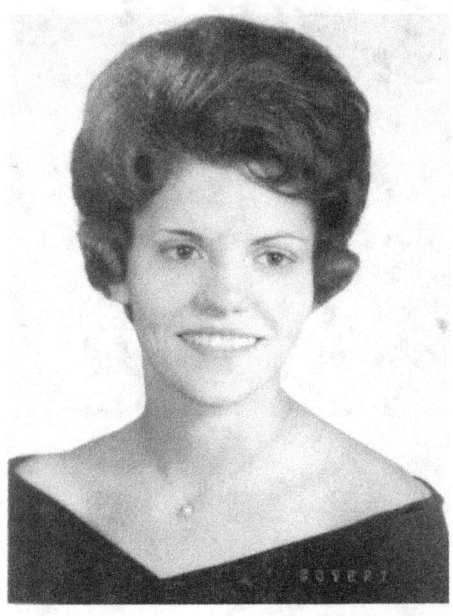

Mom's Engagement Photo taken in 1966.

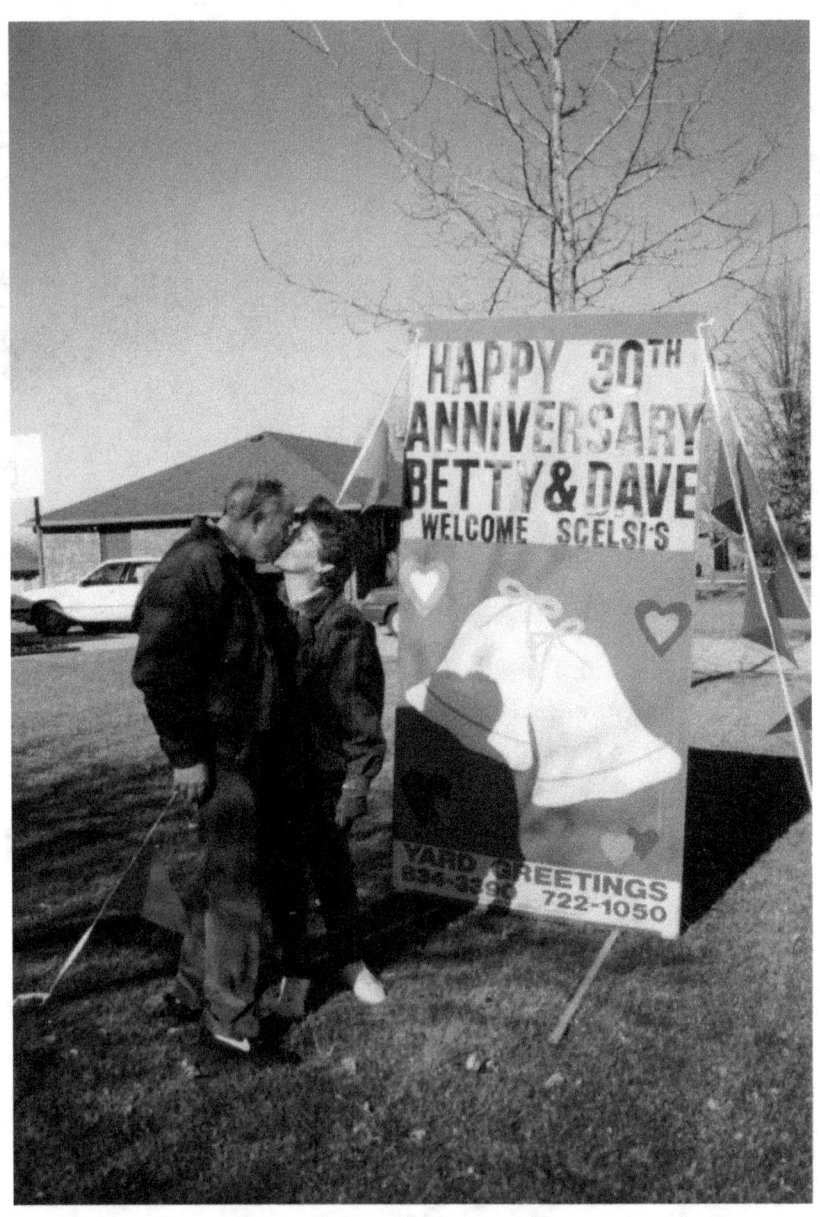

November 1996, Thanksgiving Day. Mom and Dad were married exactly on Thanksgiving Day November, 24, 1966. It was a popular day to get married then. Mom and Dad are posing in front of a sign that Sara had placed in our front yard congratulating them on their 30th anniversary and welcoming the Scelsi's who were visiting from Chicago Illinois.

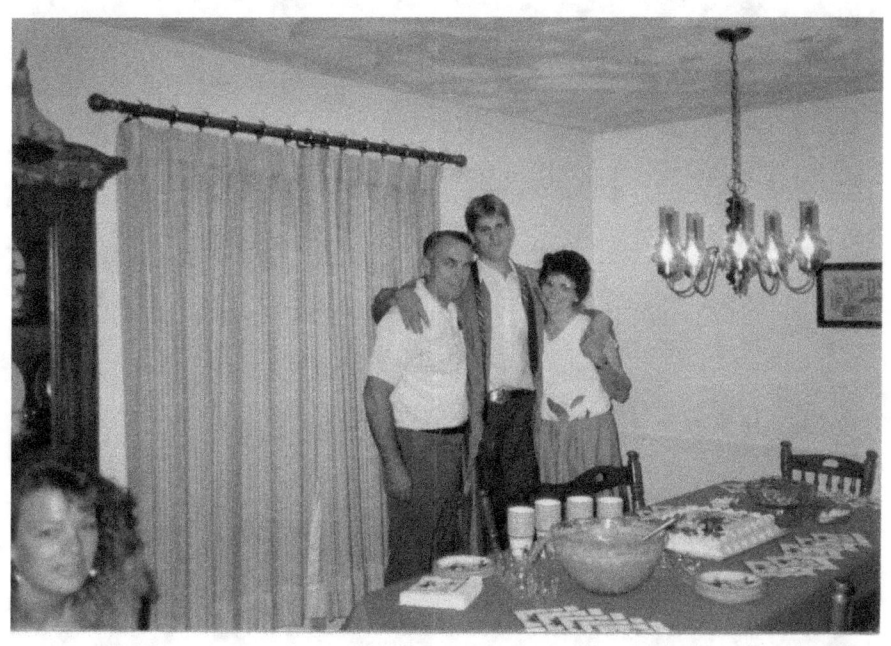

Dad, Mark, and Mom, at Mark's High School Graduation Party in May of 1987. Mom always had a beautiful spread on special occasions.

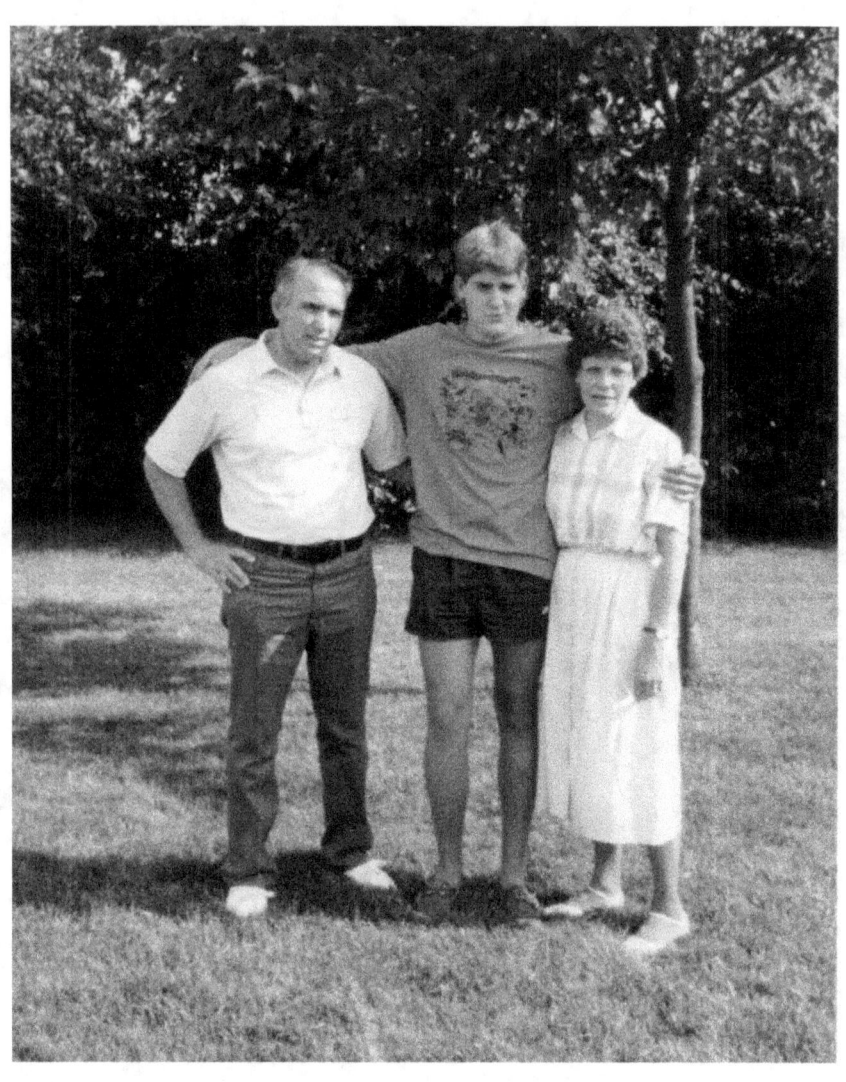

Dad, Mark, and Mom posing a week before Mark
left to join the Navy in July of 1987.

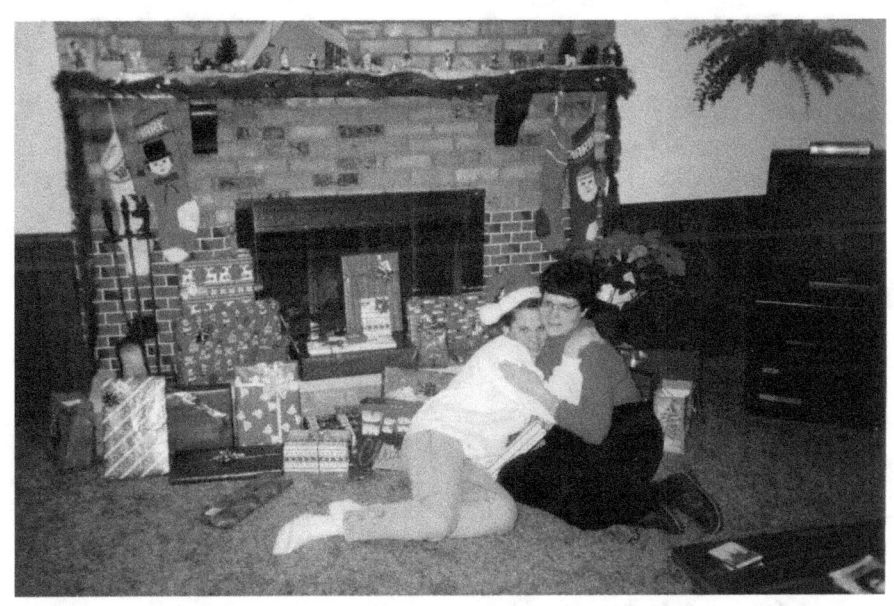

Mom and Sara celebrating Christmas in late 80's, early 90's.
Mom liked to wear a Santa hat when handing out gifts.

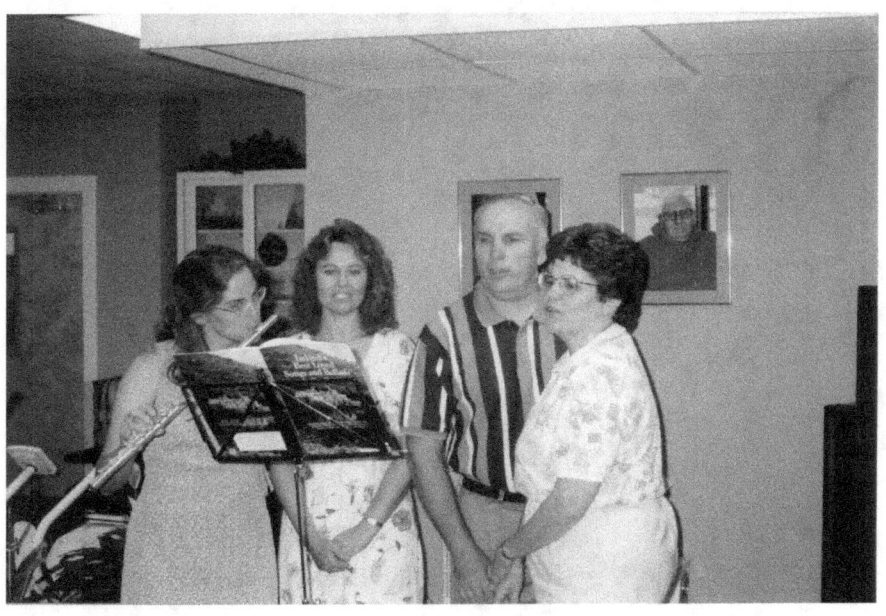

Susan playing her flute for Grandma Weber and Grandma
Cheaney at Regina Continuing Care Center, Evansville
Indiana. Susan, Aunt Judy, Dad, and Mom.

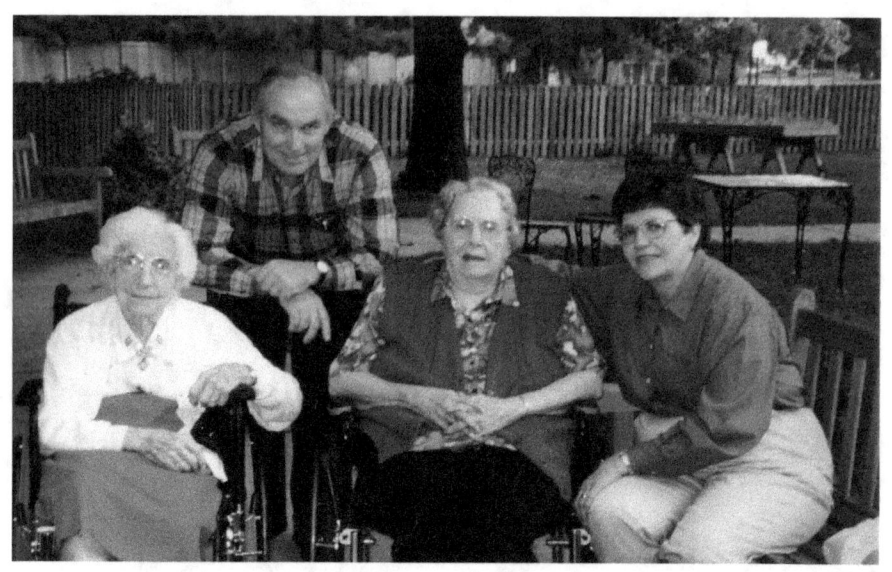

Grandma Cheaney, Dad, Grandma Weber, and Mom
visiting at Regina Continuing Care Center in Evansville
Indiana where the 2 Grandmas resided .

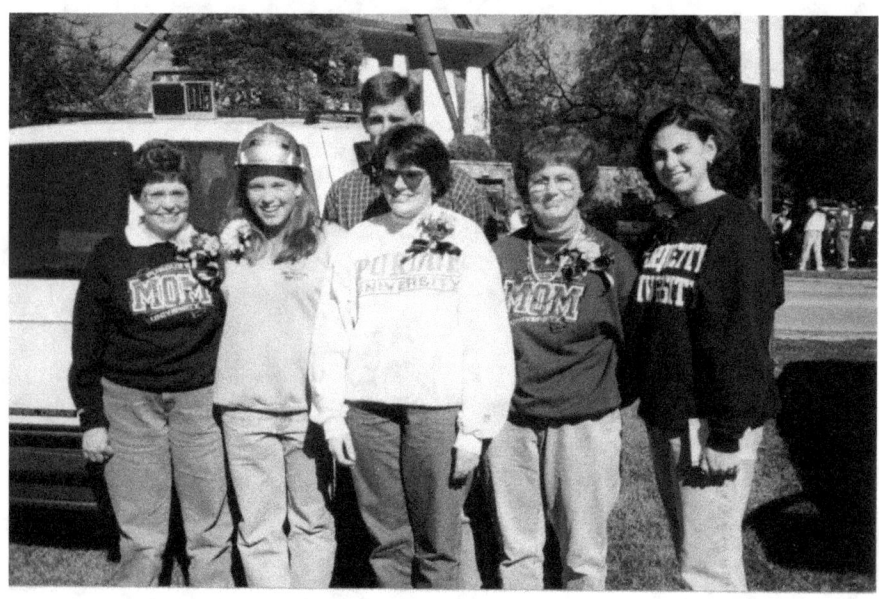

At Purdue Homecoming in September of 1996. Later that day at
Halftime, Sara would be named Purdue's Homecoming Queen. Mom,
Sara, Mark, Maria , Aunt Marian Seib, and Cousin Vicki Van Alphen.

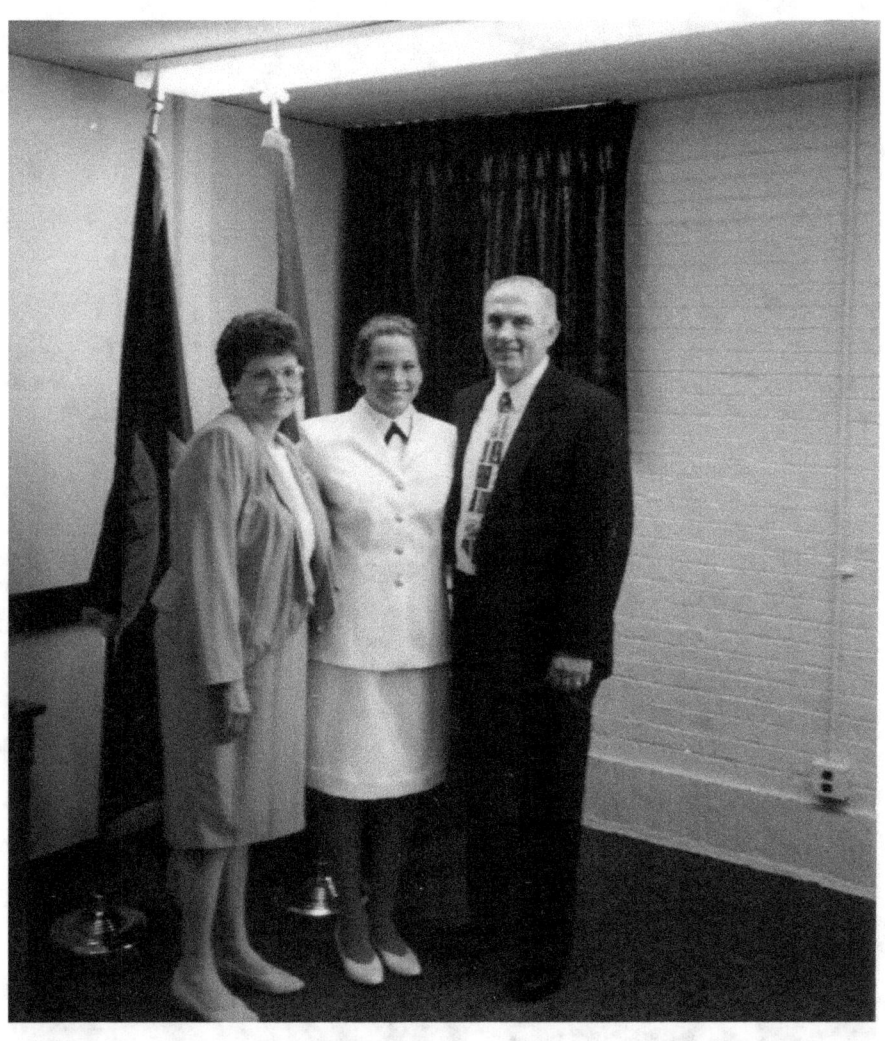

Mom, Sara, and Dad posing on Sara's Commissioning into the Navy Nurse Corp which was a proud moment for Mom and Dad in 1997.

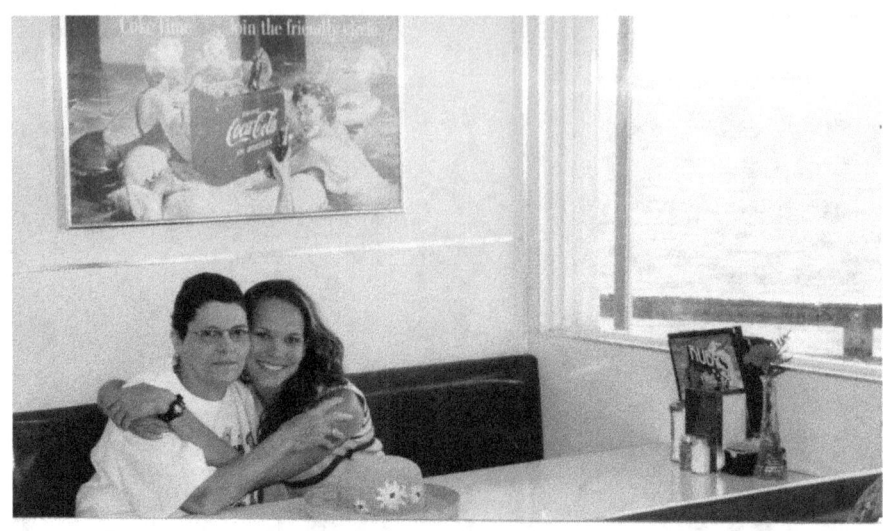

Mom and Sara in San Diego CA in June of 2001

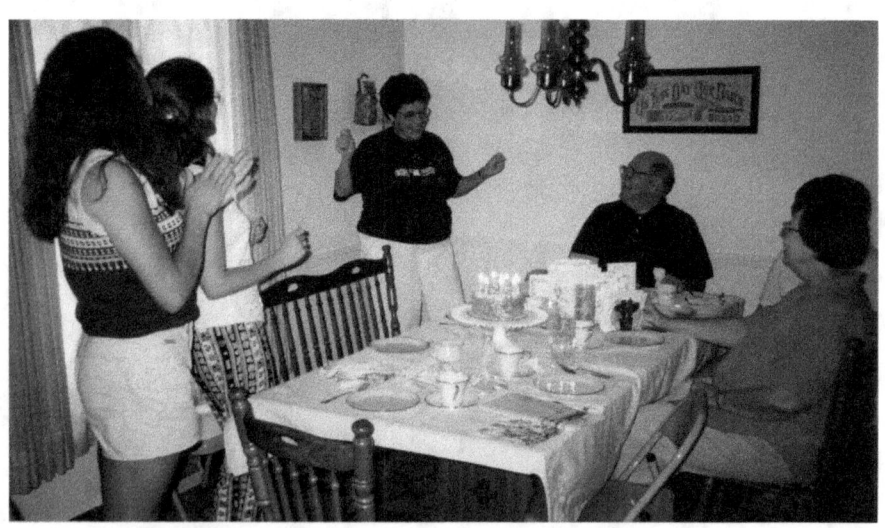

Mom demonstrating how she does the hula hoop on her
birthday in late 80's.(This tradition began when she was in
Nursing School when Mom was taught the song by a classmate)
Sara, Susan, Mom, Uncle John and Aunt Alma Higbee.

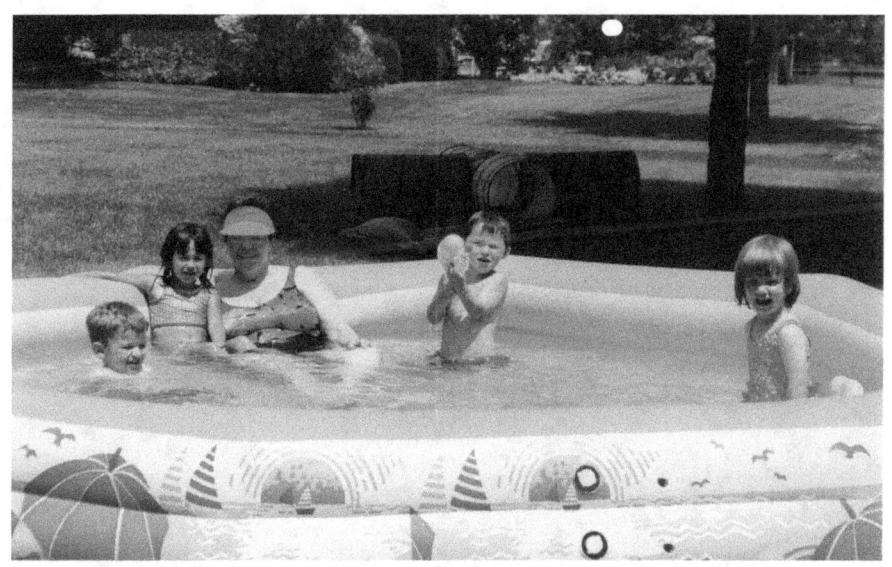

Mom wearing a pink sun visor playing with
the neighbor kids in their pool.

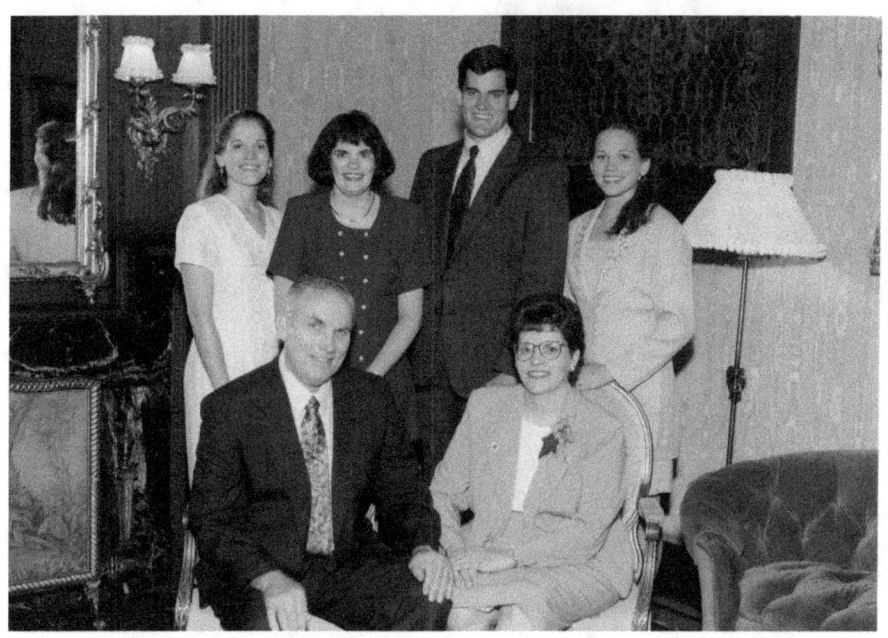

Cheaney Family Picture in July 1995 at Cousin Jen Thomas'
Wedding. Susan, Maria, Mark, Sara, Mom, and Dad.

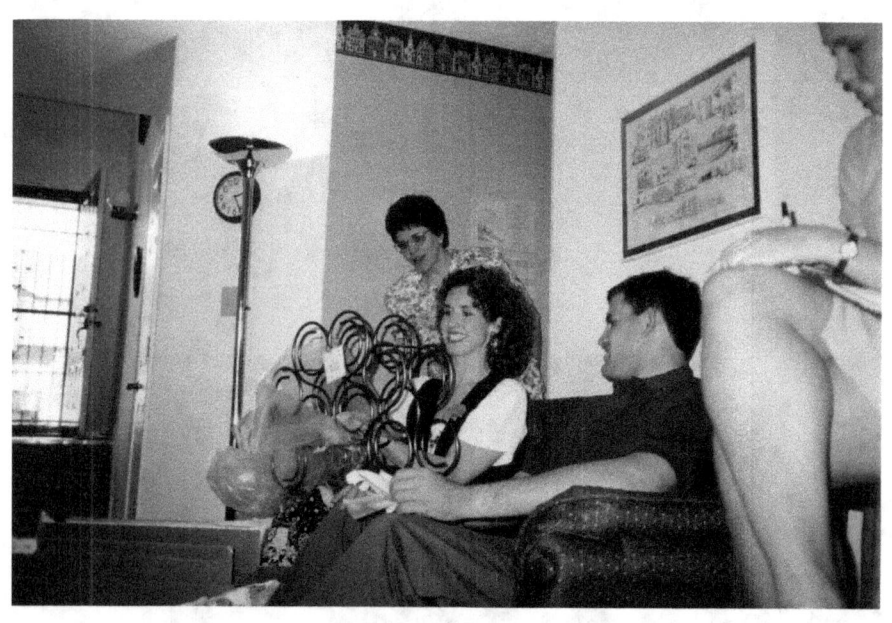

Mom having a good time at Tracy and Mark's
Bridal Shower in April of 1997.

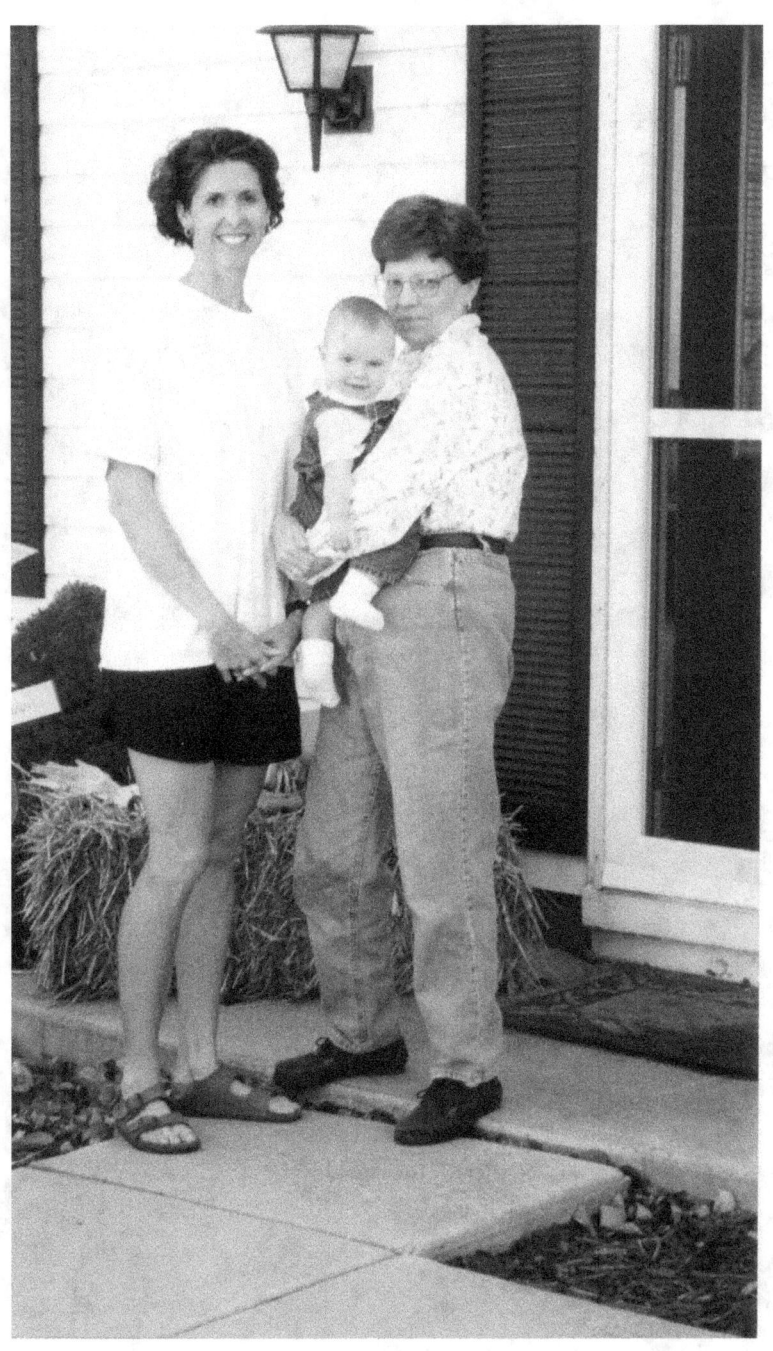

Tracy, Colin, Mom- Mom was very proud of
her first grandchild, Colin in 1999.

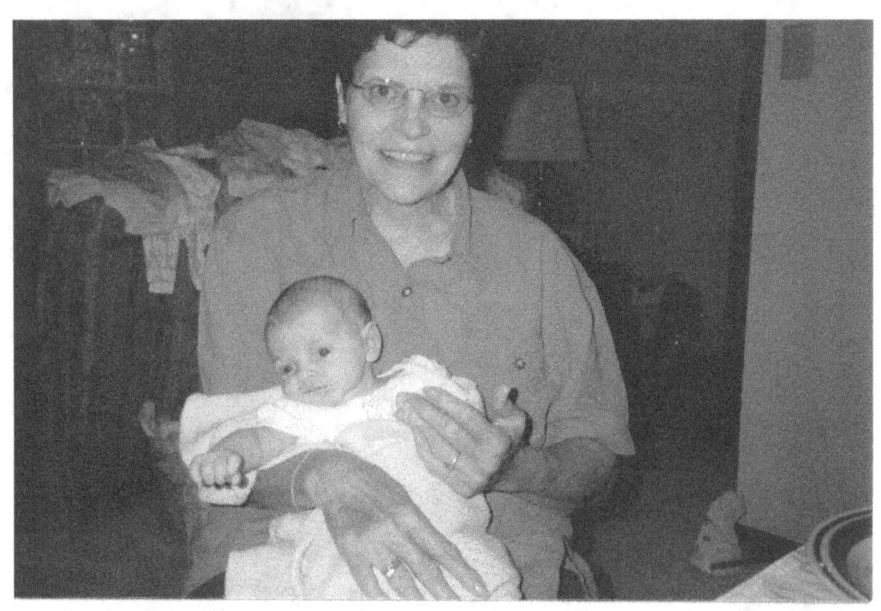

Mom holding Susan's baby girl Alma at 3 weeks of age in
June of 2001. This was Mom's first grand daughter.

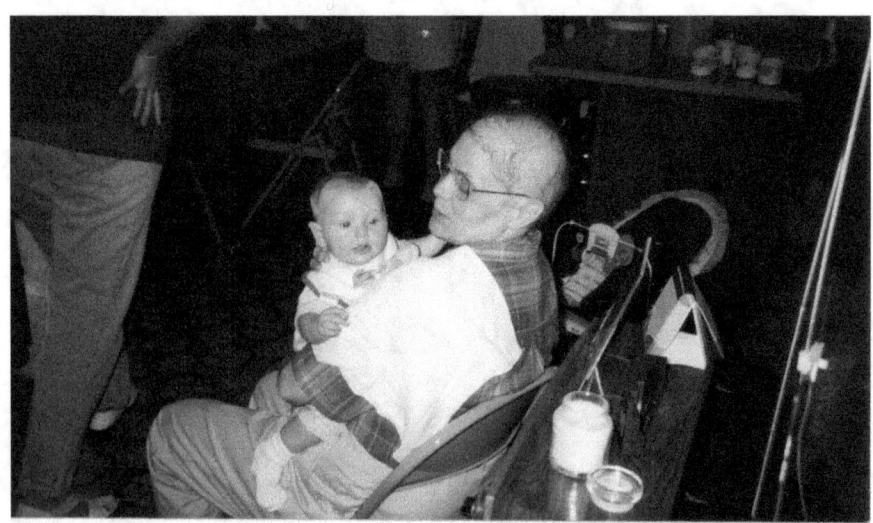

Mom holding Colin in July of 1999 after returning home from
her first hospitalization when diagnosed with Leukemia.

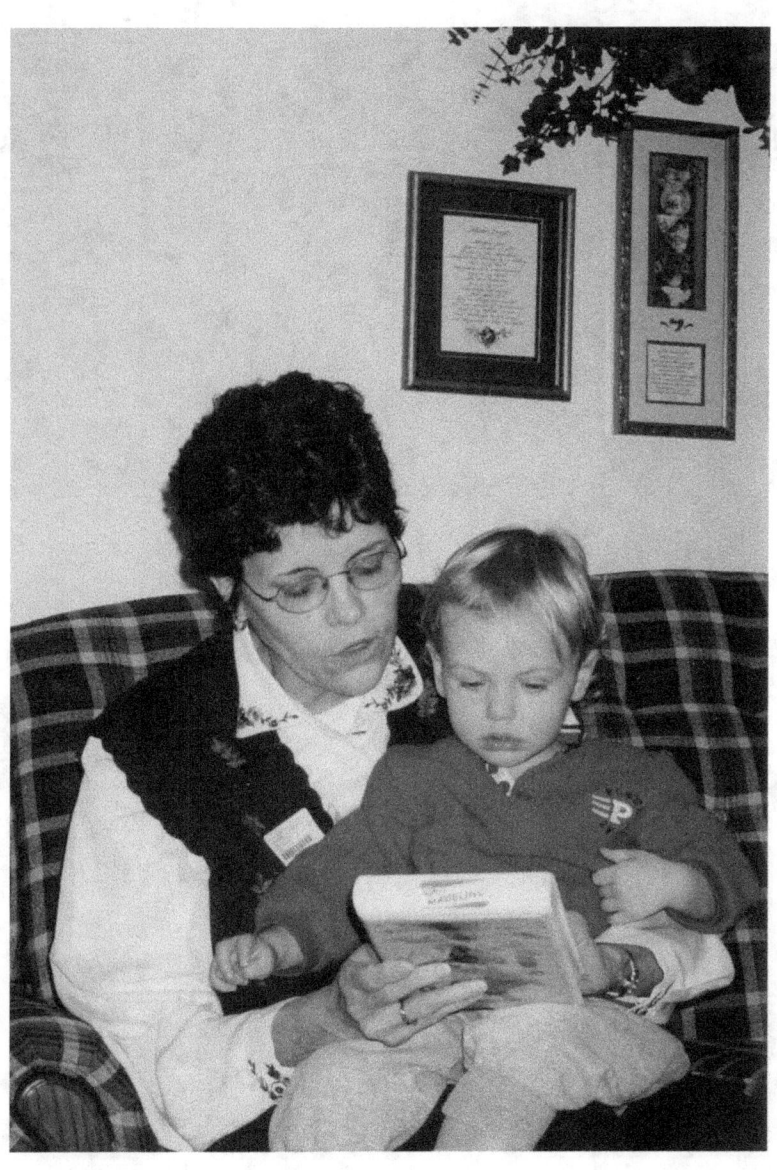

January 2001- Mom reading a book to Colin after
returning home from an outpatient hospital visit.

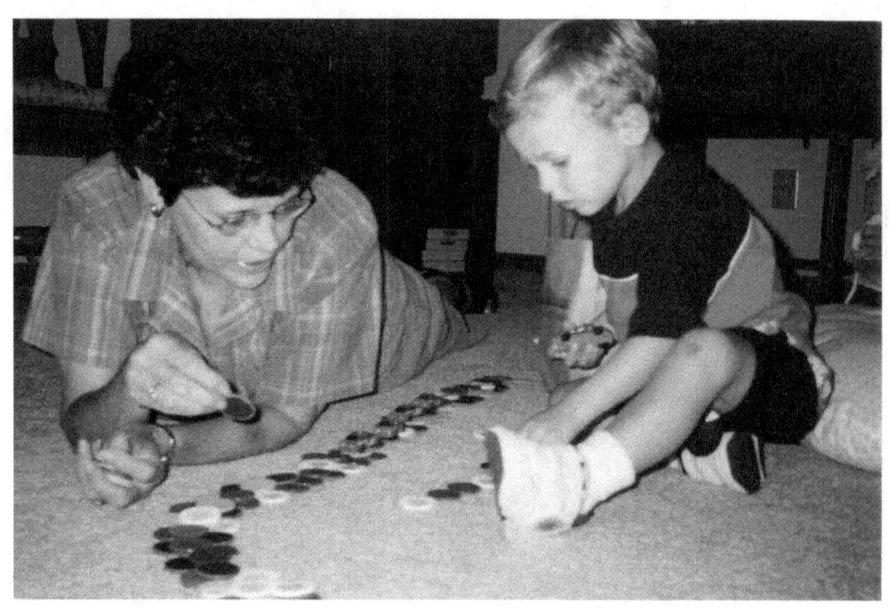

July 25, 1999- Mom with Colin playing with poker
chips that had belonged to Grandma Weber.

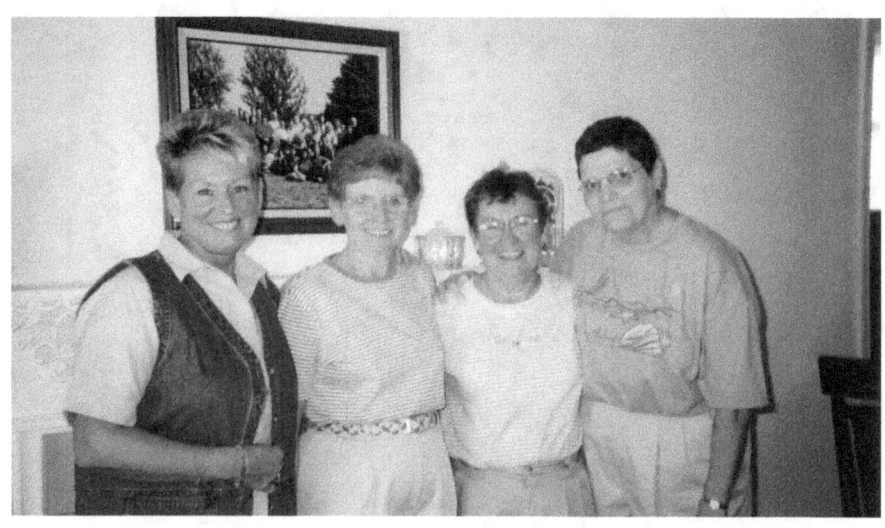

The Retired gals from Greenwood Family Practice:
Ellen McGee, Anita Upchurch, Wanda Pear, and Mom.
Missing from this picture is Shirley Kennedy.

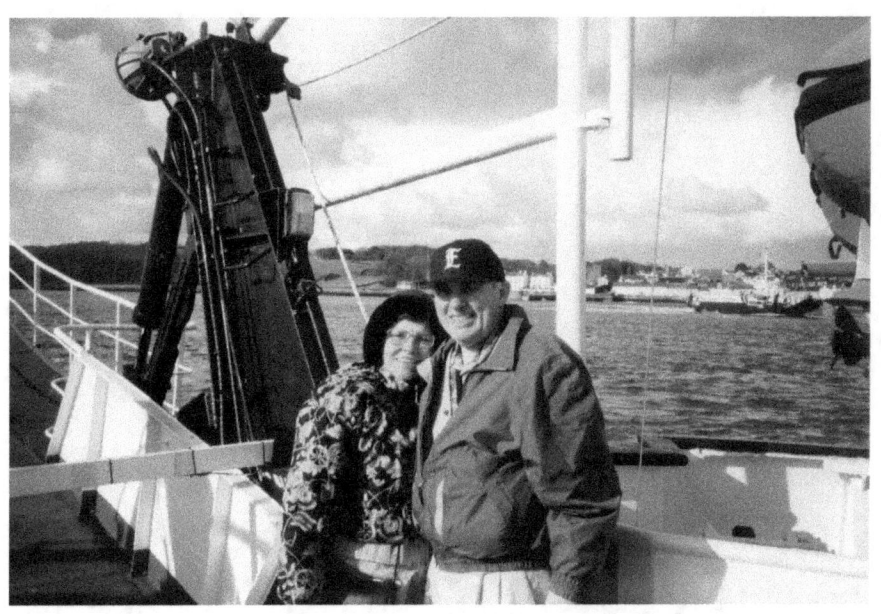

Mom and Dad on a boat ride in Europe, April 1998. So glad they took this 3 week trip as mom was diagnosed with Acute Myleoid Leukemia approximately 1 year later.

www.ingramcontent.com/pod-product-compliance
Lightning Source LLC
Chambersburg PA
CBHW071257280526
45788CB00004B/1746